Natural Penis Enlargement Guide For Men

INTRODUCTION

This Book Is All About

Natural Penis Enlargement Guide for Men,
Proven Ways, Exercises, Methods, and Tips for Increasing Your Penis Girth and Length,
Priceless Techniques for Improving Your Hardness, Love-Making Ability, Ejaculation Control.

Table of Contents

Alternative One: Stretch It Out

Your first set of exercises focuses on stretching the length, which is more than enough to get you moving in the right direction. You will be stretching not only your penis, but also the erectile tissue.

You'll want to pick just one of the four stretching exercises, so try them all out over the next few days and see which one works best for you. Switch to another if any of them cause you pain, are difficult to achieve, or do not appear to be having the desired effect in your specific case.

The first stretching exercise we'll go over is a very popular one, and it's the technique that most men credit for their success.
When you begin, your penis should be flaccid, and you can do the exercise standing or sitting down, whichever is more comfortable for you.

1. Firmly grasp the head of your penis with one hand, being careful not to cut off circulation.

2. Extend the head of your penis as far as you can without causing discomfort - and especially without causing pain.

3. Hold it in place for five minutes, using a timer to keep track. Pull the head of your penis out a little bit further after each minute. You may experience discomfort when attempting to do this, especially as you begin your penis enhancement program. If this is the case, stop pulling rather than risking injury. Continue to try until you can stretch without pain.

4. After the five minutes is up, take a full minute to relax.

5. After that, whip your penis in circles. You should make at least 30 circular motions. The goal here is to get the blood flowing again if stretching has slowed it down.

As a result, it is critical not to skip it.

6. Repeat the five-minute pull four times more, but with a slight variation for each iteration. Pull your penis in a different direction each time, whether to the left, to the right, upwards, or downwards. During a session, no direction should be repeated more than once. This ensures that you are concentrating equally on all parts of your penis and stretching it as effectively as possible. Repeat the whipping movements at least 30 times after each five-minute session.

7. Pull your penis out in front of you again and stretch it as far as you can for one minute (again, without pain or discomfort).

8. Gently pull on your penis ten times without causing pain.

9. You're done for the day; repeat this exercise tomorrow after your penis has had time to recover.

Finally, avoid putting any pressure on your dorsal nerve, which runs along the top of your penis. This will almost certainly cause pain and prevent you from reaping the benefits of the exercise.

The men who have recommended this exercise claim to have seen a difference in just two weeks and to have continued to see results for up to four months after that, resulting in several inches of growth.

Alternative Two: Stretch It Out

This stretching exercise is similar to the first one, but a little less complicated. It can be an excellent starting point if you are unsure of your technique or are not comfortable with the additional stretching required.

from Option 1. Again, your penis must be flaccid when performing this exercise, and the preparation that we discussed in the first chapter is essential.

1. Take one of your hands and grasp the head of your penis. As is always the case, your grip should be firm but not painful.

2. Extend your penis in front of you so that you can feel the stretch all the way down its shaft.

3. Hold your penis in this position for 30 seconds, then release and take some deep breaths. Repeat until you've logged at least 20 minutes of stretching, then stop for at least 20 minutes.

4. It is best to begin slowly with this exercise. Stretch your penis for five minutes at a time for the first few days, then gradually increase the amount of time you stretch during a session and the number of sessions you perform in a day.

Men who have tried this technique claim to have added up to two full inches to the length of their penis over time - if you're careful how you go about it, you can achieve the same results.

Alternative Three: Extending It

The third exercise you might want to try is stretching your penis while it is flaccid and while it is erect. You'll want it soft at first because you'll get to the hard part later.

1. Take your dominant hand and pull your penis forward and away from your body. You want to create a tugging movement before allowing it to return to its normal state.

Rep this 10 times, holding the stretch for 15 to 20 seconds each time.

2. Repeat the first step, but this time pull your penis to the right at an angle. Hold the stretch for a total of 15 to 20 seconds each time.

3. Repeat the procedure, but this time pull to the left.

4. Repeat once more, but this time pull downwards.

5. Your penis must be erect for the next steps. Rub your thumb over the tip until this happens.

6. Now, with your dominant hand's thumb and forefinger, circle the very base of your penis. Pull forward about an inch and repeat ten times. The goal is to direct all of your penis' energy upwards toward its head.

7. Pull your penis to the right and rotate it in circles with your finger and thumb while simultaneously pulling it outwards.

8. Repeat step 8 but pull your penis to the left instead of the right.

9. To complete the exercise, very gently slap your penis against each of your inner thighs ten times while pulling outwards at the same time.

Option Four: Extending It

If you have a spiritual bent, this fourth and final option may be the best fit for you. It is based on ancient Taoist teachings and incorporates spiritual elements you may or may not be familiar with. If you are, this may be the obvious exercise to help you improve your penis. If not, there's nothing stopping you from giving it a shot - you might end up enhancing more than just your trouser bulge.

1. Take a deep breath through your nose and into your throat, then swallow to push that air all the way down into your stomach.

2. As the air you inhaled enters your stomach and descends towards your abdomen, continue to push it lower until it reaches your penis.

3. Press the three middle fingers of one hand into the midpoint between your ball sack and anus at the same time. This is known as the Hui-Yin in Taoism. This will direct all of your breath's power into your penis and keep it there.

4. Return to your normal breathing pattern; your work there is complete.
At the same time, you will begin to pull your penis back and forth in order to stretch it as far as possible without causing discomfort. Repeat this 36 times, keeping your movements as rhythmical as possible at all times.

5. Because you'll need to keep your penis erect for the rest of this exercise, rub the head until you get an erection.

6. Wrap your entire hand around the base of your penis and slide it forward a full inch. This will force the breath energy you've directed into your penis up towards its head.

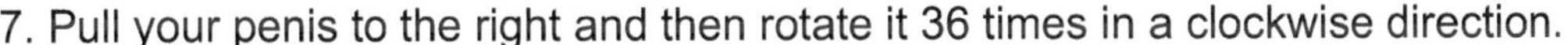

7. Pull your penis to the right and then rotate it 36 times in a clockwise direction.

8. Repeat step 8 except this time rotate your penis in the opposite direction.

9. Finally, gently slap your penis against each of your thighs 36 times.
This exercise is similar to the third option, but it includes an extra step that incorporates the power of your breath. It allows all of the energy from your body and other organs to flow downwards and enter your penis, which the Taoists believe will increase its length, tone, and, most importantly, function.

Whether you are spiritual or prefer to avoid such beliefs, the breathing component will help you relax into the rhythmic motions and successfully complete the exercise.

It's either use it or lose it.

One thing you should never forget while working on your penis enhancement program is that the more you use your penis, the better shape it will be in. Doctors and researchers are well aware that a penis can only maintain its tone and health if its muscle is regularly enriched with oxygen.

Fortunately, doing so is simple: simply keep your penis erect on a regular basis, causing a rush of blood to bring the oxygen your penis craves.
Without regular erections, your penis tissue will lose elasticity, which is bad news for your penis enhancement program. If your penis does not receive this regular oxygen infusion, it can shrink over time and lose nearly an inch in length. That's clearly counterproductive to your goals, so make sure you're getting plenty of erections.

Don't be concerned if you find yourself in a situation where your erections aren't occurring on their own, such as during a visit to your in-laws or during a period of grief. If you let it, your penis will take care of itself; all you have to do is make sure you get enough sleep. Your penis will become hard during the REM phase of sleep, which is also when you dream.
If you sleep long enough to have plenty of REM periods, your penis will do enough maintenance on its own to keep it from shortening.

Working On Width

Length is great, but the ladies always seem to say that your girth makes a difference. If you want to improve the size of your penis, the circumference should not be overlooked.

Fortunately, techniques for increasing your girth have been around for centuries, and cultures, tribes, and individuals all over the world and throughout history will attest to their effectiveness. The key is to work out your penis while it is partially erect rather than completely flaccid or completely erect.

This type of exercise is beneficial for developing the penis as a whole, so that its length and girth grow proportionally. You will also notice that the weight and density of your penis improve as you progress.

It's known as "Jelqing," which translates from Arabic to "milking," and it's widely regarded as the best and most effective natural method of enhancing your penis available. Records show that men in India, Africa, and the Middle East eventually achieved a penis length of an eye-watering 17 inches - and they weren't born with those proportions.

The techniques are also popular in the Western world, and most men who try them report several inches of growth in a year - one man from California even doubled his penis size in that time.

It works by forcing blood into your penis, which causes the spaces within your penis to gradually increase in volume, allowing them to hold more blood while erect. At the same time, you'll be improving your penis' health, increasing its strength, and making it bigger.

When performing milking exercises, keep the following safety precautions in mind: Never perform any of these exercises while fully erect.

This can be extremely damaging to the veins in your penis, with long-term consequences.

Unless otherwise instructed, always use lubricant for these exercises. If you don't, you'll at best be sore at the end of your session, and at worst, you may injure yourself permanently.

Shower Time - Working On Width

Before we begin your girth exercises, let's go over the history of these techniques and the special preparation that has always been used to enhance their effects. You, too, can incorporate a variation of this ancient secret into your daily routine, and the results are frequently described as incredible.

Throw out your shower gel and replace it with ancient wisdom; you won't be sorry.
The Arabs, who are famous around the world for their penis size and strength, have been practicing milking exercises for centuries. The work begins when a boy is only six years old. A boy learns from his father that stroking his penis slowly from the base all the way to the tip will increase its size and length over time. He begins to follow this practice in a ritualistic manner, devoting half an hour to it each day.

Wealthy boys are eventually sent to a special establishment where the attendant will strip him naked and massage his penis with an oil preparation. The goal is to relax all of his muscles while also increasing his sexual stimulation.

The oil blend is thought to be the technique's secret ingredient, so you might want to make your own version to use while working through your enhancement program. As you begin, you should be near a shower.

1. Combine a heaping tablespoon of white or yellow corn meal mix with a quart of pure mayonnaise to make the blend.

2. Cover your hair with a shower cap and then apply the oil blend all over your body, beginning at the top of your head and neck and working your way down. Cover your entire body, from head to toe.

3. Stand in the shower with the water running hot, but do not wash your hair.

Place your feet directly in the stream. You will first take advantage of the steam produced by the shower.

4. Apply the mixture to your skin in circular motions, slowly and methodically. If you prefer, you can work on your face with a cloth.

5. Adjust the temperature of your shower to a more comfortable level and allow the water to rinse the oil blend from your skin. As you do so, you will feel a tingling sensation all over your body.

When your shower is finished, the results will be breathtaking. Not only will you be tingling, but your skin will have a glow and satin sheen unlike anything you've ever seen before, and you'll feel uplifted and joyful while remaining completely relaxed. When combined with the milking exercises discussed in the following chapter, this shower technique can be an excellent addition to your routine.

Alternative One - Working On Width

Your first option is a very simple technique that you should practice five days a week. The end result should be a three-inch increase in length and a proportional increase in girth. Be aware that it is common for men who try this technique to become discouraged during the first month because you are unlikely to see any specific results. However, by the second month, you will begin to see exactly what you were hoping for.

1. Apply lubricant to your penis and store it somewhere easy to reach - you may need to apply more during the exercise.

2. Squeeze the base of your penis between your thumb and forefinger, then pull up towards the tip while pushing your penis downwards. This is intended to make your penis semi-erect, so stop as soon as it does.

Remember, never perform this exercise on a fully erect penis.
3. Form a circle with your thumb and forefinger and tightly grip the base of your penis, then sweep downwards and outwards in one long sweep.

4. Immediately repeat the motion with your other hand on the base of your penis, carrying the stroke through from the base to the tip.

5. Repeat this process, swapping hands so that you're making a rhythmic milking motion. You should move your hands over every part of your penis except the tip of the head, and you should remain semi-erect throughout. If you feel yourself becoming fully hard, either stop for a few moments to allow it to subside or squeeze a little harder - whichever works best for you.

6. Continue until you have completed between 200 and 300 strokes.

at medium pressure, which will take around 10 minutes.

7. For the second week, increase the strength of your strokes slightly and continue until you have performed between 300 and 500 strokes, which will take approximately 15 minutes.

8. From the third week onwards, you can spend 20 minutes a day performing this exercise, completing 500 or more strokes with as much pressure as you can stand without discomfort. Add more lubricant as you need to, never allowing your penis to become dry as this will lead to some seriously unpleasant irritation exactly where you'd rather not experience it.

9. As you finish, encourage the circulation in your penis to return to normal by slapping it up and down around 30 times.

This technique is very much an exercise in self-control. As you stroke your penis, it's only natural that you will feel your excitement levels increase – that's how it's meant to work, after all. You will need to pause or squeeze to stop this from happening so that you can complete the exercise while still only semi-erect.

Alternative Two: Working On Width

This method of milking is widely thought to have astounding effects on width and overall size, so if it suits your technique, it's an excellent choice. Again, make sure your penis is lubricated before beginning the exercise, and stay semi-erect at all times - it won't work if you're fully erect or soft, and it can sometimes be harmful.

1. With your penis semi-erect and lubrication all over it, rub a little more lubricant between your palms.

2. Form a circle with your forefinger and thumb and tightly grip the base of your penis. Maintain this grip throughout the next stage.

3. Slide your hand all the way down your penis until it reaches the head, then pull. During the process, you will notice that the head of your penis grows larger.

4. Repeat the previous two steps with your other hand right away.

5. Return to your first hand as soon as the second reaches the head of your penis. Continue at a relatively quick pace. If you feel yourself approaching a climax, stop and wait for the urge to pass.

During the first few weeks of working with this exercise, limit yourself to no more than 200 repetitions in a single session. This should take about 10 minutes in total, and you should stop if you feel any soreness or discomfort. You can always start again in a few minutes after you've rested, but if your penis is still sore, you should wait a day or so.

After you've been using this technique for two weeks, start increasing the number of repetitions. Finally, you can incorporate

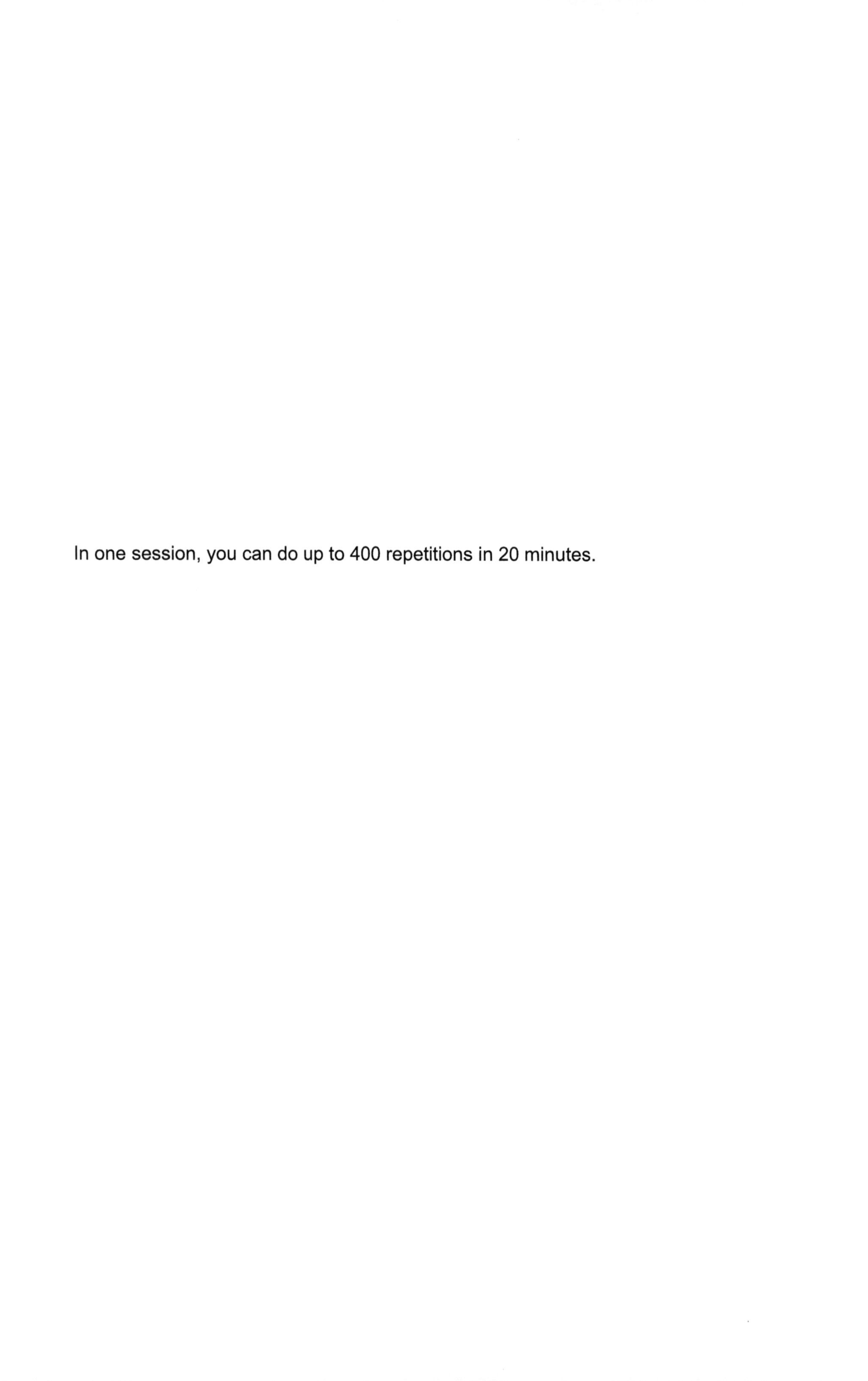

In one session, you can do up to 400 repetitions in 20 minutes.

Alternative Three: Working On Width

The third exercise option for improving your girth and overall penis strength differs slightly from the previous two. You should be more gentle with this exercise than you were with the others, and you should be aware that it will cause the head of your penis to turn very red and swell more than you might expect. Don't be alarmed; this is a normal reaction to the exercise; you're forcing a lot of blood into the head of your penis, which is what causes the color change. Of course, there should be no discomfort involved, and you should stop immediately if you begin to feel any pain.

1. While the penis shaft is still soft, apply lubricant all the way down it.

2. With your thumb and first finger, stretch your penis downward and slightly to one side.

3. Repeat with your other hand, pulling your penis to the opposite side.

4. Continue to repeat with one hand then the other to create a milking action. Be gentle at first, but once you've reached a semi-erect position, you can increase the force you're using simultaneously.

Repeat the technique 100 times over the first few days, then gradually increase the repetitions. You should eventually be able to complete 200 repetitions without any discomfort.

Alternative Four: Working On Width

This technique is designed specifically for men who want to increase the size of their penis head. It's essentially the same as the first girth-improvement technique you tried, but with a lot less speed and force. Some refer to it as the Tao technique.

1. Apply lubricant, then use all of your fingers on one hand to push blood up into the head of your penis. This will apply some pressure, which should be held for about 10 seconds before releasing.

2. Squeeze the shaft during the motion if you want the blood to engorge in the head of your penis.

3. Let go of the squeeze and rest for a few seconds before repeating. You can repeat this as many times as you want, but never for more than 10 minutes at a time.
This exercise will eventually allow the head of your penis to take in more blood by expanding its capacity. This will give your penis a bell-shaped end.

Alternative Five - Working On Width

Your final girth exercise option is the only one that does not require lubrication. This is useful if you have five minutes to spare but are unable to reach the lube bottle. Some men say it's also a great technique to use in the mornings, right after waking up from a night's sleep. It can be done while you're still in bed without making a mess, and it's also the time of day when your testosterone levels are at their highest, so many people believe it's the best time to work on improving your penis.

Simply follow the steps in either the first or second exercise option to perform the dry milking technique. This time, however, you will not be using lubricant, so you will not want to slide your fingers over your skin for many repetitions. Instead, squeeze and pull your penis skin but do not slide.

If there is too much area to cover in a single stroke, you can work on the base of your penis first, followed by the head end. If you start to feel sore, stop immediately and rest for at least a day before ccontinuing

Introducing Kegel Exercises for Penis Control

A larger and thicker penis is great, but enhancing your penis requires another factor. You will be able to maintain much more powerful erections for a longer period of time if you strengthen your Kegel muscle. It will also increase the intensity of your orgasms, and some men report that after working on this muscle for a while, they are able to achieve multiple orgasms.
But that's not all. You will also gain more control over your ejaculations and reduce the amount of time it takes to recover between orgasms. Kegel exercises can even help your prostate's health.

The Kegel muscle is actually another name for the pubococcygeal muscles, which run from your pubic bone to your tailbone. Press the area just behind your testicles if you want to feel it. This is the muscle that controls urination, but it is also the one that causes orgasm and causes your ejaculation to pump. It is present in both men and women, and you may have had a previous experience with the pleasure it can provide - if your partner has ever rubbed this area during a blow or hand job, or even during sex, you will have noticed how intense the results can be.
It's called the Kegel region because the exercises to strengthen these muscles were named after a gynecologist named Arnold Kegel, who discovered how to strengthen them - and the benefits of doing so - back in the 1950s. He discovered that contracting the muscles in a controlled manner improved them in the same way that lifting weights increases the size and strength of your pecs and biceps.

Women have been taught this secret for years and know that it is the best way to enhance their sexual pleasure, but men are much less likely to be aware of, let alone know how to strengthen, their Kegel muscles. Men, ironically, have an easier time locating the muscle in question and performing exercises to strengthen it. In the following chapters, we'll show you how to find it and then explain how to work it - and with these exercises, you'll notice a difference in just a few days.

Penis Control: Where Are Your Kegels?

The first step in improving your penis control is, of course, identifying your Kegel muscle. You'll be able to flex and release it consciously once you know where it is and how it feels.
Stop your urine in the middle of the stream the next time you visit the little boy's room. That muscle you're tensing to keep it in place? This is your Kegel muscle.

Repeat the exercise after releasing the stream for a few seconds. Take note of how easily you can completely stop the flow. At first, you may not be able to stop it completely and may only be able to reduce the flow slightly. However, as you exercise the muscle, your ability to stop the urine midstream will improve incrementally until you can pretty much hold it completely for as long as you want.

As it happens, stopping your urination is more than just a good way to locate the muscle. It's also the simplest way to keep your Kegels in shape. Make a habit of stopping and starting your urine on every bathroom trip. Try it at least five times and gradually increase the time you can hold it.

Count how many seconds you can hold it for each time and see how it improves. The tightness with which you can clench will improve as well, and you should eventually be able to stop your urine flow completely.

This is a trick that women have been using for years - some women claim they can hold that muscle in place almost indefinitely, and there's no reason why you can't achieve the same level of strength.

You can also experiment with flexing it quickly and frequently. This can be easier to do, especially at first, than simply holding the muscle tight for an extended period of time.

Kegel Exercises for Penis Control

Exercising your Kegels does not have to be limited to bathroom visits.
Unlike your work to increase the length and girth of your penis, you can exercise this muscle at any time and in any place. Nobody can see what you're doing, so you can do your exercises while sitting at your desk or riding the train.

There are only a few times during the day when you won't be able to work on your Kegel muscle. It is critical to exercise it on a regular basis, so try to do at least one set of these exercises every day. You can vary the type of exercise you do as much as you want, as long as you work on your Kegels every day. Here are some alternatives for you to consider:
Contract and release the muscle quickly and with control.

Begin by doing this for a set of 20 contractions, but gradually increase the number. You should eventually be able to do at least 100 in a single session - some men can do 250 at once. Work your way up to being able to perform a total of 1000 contractions per day for the best results.
Contract the muscle and hold it for as long as you can.

This may only be for a few seconds at first. As you practice, you should be able to hold the muscle in place for 30 seconds or more, increasing its strength and endurance.
Flex and then release your Kegel muscle for two seconds. Repeat as many times as you can, increasing the number of times you can do in a single session.

Flex your muscle to its full tautness as slowly as you can and then immediately relax. As you get better at this technique, you'll notice that your muscles flutter as you let go of the tension, which can be very relaxing.

Push the muscle outwards, just as you would when squeezing the last drops of urine out. This exercise should not be performed when you need to use the restroom because it can cause your anus to open, which can be problematic if you are not paying attention to your timing.

As your muscles improve in health and strength, you will notice many changes in your sexual enjoyment - but some of these changes will be subtle. You'll thank yourself later for those, though. Your Kegel muscles can help you maintain erections for longer periods of time, even if you're having difficulty doing so - many doctors recommend these exercises for erection problems.

These exercises will boost your arousal, prolong and enhance your orgasms, and increase the amount of time you last during sex. And, as your body ages, it can help you avoid incontinence because your muscles will remain firm and tight. When you combine this with the possibility of multiple orgasms and the ability to postpone your ejaculation, you'll wonder why you didn't start these exercises years ago.

Finalizing Touches

When it comes to your penis enhancement program, the end is just as important as the beginning. After you've finished all of your exercises, you should devote some love and attention to this most sensitive area to ensure that it doesn't suffer long-term consequences.

Begin this final stage by gently massaging your penis to restore normal blood flow and work out any kinks that have formed. If you want, you can buy enlargement creams with herbal, natural ingredients for a smoother massage, but the real work in this program has already been done.

Next, use the same hot compress that you used to begin your exercise program. This will help to stimulate your cells to repair themselves if you have inadvertently caused damage with your actions, and it will help to relax it and stimulate new cell growth if you have not.

You are now ready to go about your day, confident that you have taken a significant step toward a healthier, larger, and more effective penis.

The Positive, Negative, and Negative

You may have read this book so far expecting to see mention of surgical procedures and devices that are frequently touted as having a significant impact on the size of your package. Some of them are worth mentioning, so we'll go over them in this chapter, but for the most part, they're superfluous.

If you started your regime expecting quick results and simply can't wait a couple of months for your exercise regime to kick in, you may be tempted to boost the results with one of the techniques you've seen advertised. Should you, however?

Surgical Techniques: We strongly advise against investing your money in a procedure to enlarge your penis. Not only will the extra they add be completely insensitive, doing nothing to improve your sex life, but there is a lot that can go horribly wrong. Do you really want to jeopardize your favorite body part's health and well-being for a few extra inches? There are several surgical treatments available, and while they all appear to be excellent at first glance, you will almost certainly change your mind after speaking with a doctor. According to studies, most men have no desire to proceed with surgery once they've been given a thorough explanation of the outcome, associated risks, and potential complications. A small penis is preferable to no penis at all.

Pumps for the penis: You've probably seen these devices in a variety of shapes and sizes, some with manual pumps and others with motorized pumps. The basic idea is to create a partial vacuum around your penis, causing it to engorge by drawing blood into the shaft. The pressure within the blood vessels rises as the vacuum rises. Unfortunately, studies have shown that penis pumps are not only ineffective, but also extremely harmful. A six-month study of nearly 40 men revealed a total increase of less than a millimeter. Some men claimed to be pleased with their progress, but this was attributed to the placebo effect - there was no real, physical improvement.

Penis pumps can have tangible benefits in certain situations, such as when used in conjunction with a tourniquet ring to create an erection for a man suffering from impotence or to treat Peyronie's disease, which causes the penis to curve and shorten. But it's unlikely to help the average man with an average penis. Using one for an extended period of time can cause blood vessels to burst, blisters to form, and make you wish you'd left it in the packaging.

Clamping is a homemade technique used by some men that is as painful and dangerous as it sounds. Clamping attempts to enlarge your penis by constricting the base for an extended period of time in order to prevent blood from flowing back out of it. If you've ever sat on your hand for too long and felt numbness and pins and needles, you know how unpleasant this is likely to be in your crotch region. Cable clamps, shoe strings, and cock rings are among the most commonly used implements, all of which are extremely dangerous, especially the latter. When a metal device is used to trap blood in the penis, it can become difficult to remove.

If the ring cannot be sawed off, your penis may need to be amputated. Even if the damage isn't as severe, the negative effects of clamping are frequently permanent.

Popping Pills: There is little evidence that any of the supplements on the market have any effect on penis size. We don't recommend taking pills that could disrupt your body's overall balance, especially if they're unlikely to result in the penis enlargement you seek. Because most of these penis enhancement pills are herbal in nature rather than containing chemical compounds, they are safer than their predecessors from 20 years ago. If you want to supplement your exercise program with these substances, by all means do so - but we're willing to bet that the results you're seeing are entirely due to your regimen and have little to do with the herbs.

The Young Weight Lifter: We've heard horror stories about men who thought attaching weights to their penis would help them get in shape. True, any body part will eventually stretch if

There's a brick hanging from it, but the experience won't be enjoyable. Even if you succeed, you're unlikely to retain the same level of sensitivity once you're done, and there will be plenty of negative consequences if you don't.

In general, if you want to stay healthy and keep your penis in the best possible condition, we recommend avoiding all of these techniques. Continue with the exercises; you'll thank us later.

Changing Your Way of Life

You may be surprised to find a chapter on lifestyle changes in a book about penis enhancement, but it is critical that you make a few changes to your diet and daily routine if you want to see success. Even if you're skeptical about the ability of a broccoli stem to increase the size of your package, keep in mind that a healthy body full of energy is one that has the stamina to make the most of the improvements you achieve through your exercise regimen. What are you afraid of losing?

To begin, there are some foods that you should include in your daily diet, making sure to consume at least one portion every day. These are the foods:

Milk
Yummy sweet potatoes
Salmon
Tuna
Broccoli Liver Eggs
Bananas
Onions

Why? Because the majority of these foods contain vasodilators, which relax the muscles in the walls of your blood vessels. Your blood flow in that area affects penis enhancement and the strength of your erections in general, so choose foods that can help you out. These foods have the potential to increase your penis girth, but only slightly. The most important reason to eat them is to increase the effectiveness of your exercises.

During a penis enhancement program, salmon is your go-to food.

It's high in essential fatty acids, such as omega 3. These thin your blood and improve circulation, which is essential for achieving strong and long-lasting erections.
Onions have a similar effect in increasing blood circulation, which means that more blood and oxygen are flowing through your penis.

when you really need it.
Bananas are also an important part of the diet of any man who has ever gained penis circumference. According to studies, having a healthy heart is strongly linked to having a successful penis enhancement, and the potassium in this fruit can help you achieve that. They will also lower your sodium levels, which will benefit your heart health even more.
In general, choose foods that will increase blood flow, allowing you to maintain stiffer erections for a longer period of time. Choose lean meats, fruits and vegetables, and whole grains over processed foods and junk food.

There are also herbs that you might want to try as tinctures, pills, or teas. Each will have its own positive effect and contribute to the success of your program:
Muira Pauma Bark Extract: Discovered by Amazonian shamans in Brazil, this herb stimulates arousal and combats fatigue. Simultaneously, it relaxes the corpus cavernosa in your penis, increasing its ability to engorge.

Catuaba Bark Extract: Another Brazilian herb, this plant is known for its ability to induce deep relaxation while also improving peripheral circulation and sexual abilities.

Hawthorn Berry: This small tree has a special secret: it can help you keep an erection longer and increase the sensation of your penis. Both are beneficial in the short term, but the long-term effects will also benefit your penis enhancement program. Because of its high bioflavonoid content, hawthorn berry has long been used to treat irregular heartbeats and soften arteries. These help to strengthen your blood vessels, which is an important step toward getting more blood through them.

Ali Tongkat: This herb can help you increase the size of your penis as well as your testosterone levels. It stimulates cells in your testicles, causing them to grow larger, while also increasing your penis girth and sperm count. It's probably the most popular herb for penis enlargement and a fantastic herb to include in your regimen.

of your enhancement program.
Remember that diet alone will not increase the size of your penis, and adding herbs or supplements to your diet will not result in long-term change.

However, incorporating them into a comprehensive regimen can enhance the effects of the exercises you are performing. Meanwhile, make sure to get plenty of rest so that your penis has plenty of time to harden and flood itself with the oxygen it requires. These factors, when combined, will allow you to see results much faster than you would otherwise.

Speed Workout

Not every day includes enough hours to devote one to your penis enhancement program, but you will find that results come faster and better if you are regular in your workouts. On those days that you are busy, distracted or simply too tired to concentrate on your exercises, there is an alternative you can try instead.

We don't recommend using a speed workout as your sole penis enhancement practice, but there's very little harm in including it in your overall program when you don't have the time for a full set of exercises. At the very least it will help you maintain the progress you have already made along your journey. At best, some men claim it has increased their penis length by over an inch in a few months, even without combining it with other techniques.

You may want to start out by lubricating your penis for this one, although you will still be able to complete the exercise if you've taken a five minute bathroom break at the office and you don't have any lubrication to hand.

1. Sit on the edge of a comfortable chair and use your forefinger and thumb to create a circle wrapped around the base of your penis.

2. Stroke your penis from the base all the way up to the head. Keep your grip as firm as possible without causing discomfort and try as best you are able to stretch out the skin as you go.

3. When you reach the end, start again at the base. Keep repeating the motion and, every time you do, squeeze just that little bit more tightly. This will keep the blood trapped in your penis. Increase

your speed with every iteration.

4. Somewhere along the way, you will inevitably start to feel your penis becoming erect. Allow it to do so and keep going until you are fully hard.

5. Move back to the base and hold it tightly with one hand. With the

Create a similar grip at the opposite end, towards the tip.

6. Using both hands, stretch out your penis as far as possible without causing pain.

7. Push your penis to the right and hold it there for ten seconds.

8. Pull your penis straight out and hold it there for 10 seconds.

9. Push your penis to the left and hold it there for 10 seconds.

Finally, push it down and hold it for 10 seconds.
11. Repeat the previous four steps four times more, then release your grip on the base of your penis. You will immediately feel the blood start to flow and will be able to ejaculate if necessary. A speed workout only takes about five minutes out of your day, which isn't too difficult to find even during the busiest of weeks. You can also do the exercise up to three times in one day.

However, take care not to completely cut off circulation to your penis while performing this exercise - this is an unhealthful situation. This technique should never cause you any discomfort, so if you do, it means you're doing something wrong. It is always preferable to use lubricant, and it is critical to avoid stretching too much at once.

The goal of this speed workout is to target your erectile tissue, and doing so will create tension by stretching the skin. This means that incorporating a speed workout into your routine has advantages beyond simply increasing penis length. It will increase skin elasticity while also expanding the space inside the chambers of your penis, known as the corpora cavernosa. If you're wondering how useful having extra air pockets can be, consider this: the more blood you can fill these spaces with, the larger the overall mass of your penis while it's erect. That is a penis enhancement in and of itself.

Putting Everything Together

You've tried the exercises, decided which ones you like best, and made sure to follow all of the safety and health precautions along the way. You're satisfied with the elements of the penis enhancement regime you've narrowed down to this point, so there's only one thing left to do: put it all together.

In this chapter, we'll show you how to turn these exercises into a daily routine that you can stick to. You can modify the regimen to include exercises that are simple to perform, do not cause pain or discomfort, and fit into your busy schedule. You can also vary your program by switching between exercises on a daily, weekly, or monthly basis. The more variety you include, all pointing to the same overall goals, the more even your development will be and the less likely you will become bored.

Include the following items in your program:
1. Hot Compress Introduction: 5 minutes - Regardless of the other exercises you do, this is a must. Always begin by properly preparing your penis.

2. Stretch It Out Exercise: 30 minutes - Begin your workout with one of the stretching exercises from the first few chapters.

Depending on the exercise, you may not want to spend the full 30 minutes on this section at first, but you should aim to gradually increase your time.

3. Interval: 1 minute - After your first exercise session, gently whip your penis around 30 times. As you do so, make sure to cup your testicles in your other hand to prevent them from flying around and injuring themselves.

4. Working on Width Exercise: 20 minutes - Select your preferred option from the Working on Width chapters to incorporate a girth-increasing exercise into your routine. Again, start with a lower number than 20 minutes and gradually increase to the maximum.

Remember that this section requires a semi-erect penis at all times, and you must resist the urge to ejaculate

.

5. Penis Control Exercises: 5 Minutes - At this point in your regimen, choose a Kegel exercise and perform it for at least five minutes.
It's included here partly to round out your program and partly to remind you that this essential exercise should be part of your daily routine. You can include your control exercises at other points in your daily schedule if you want to include other or the same Kegel exercises during the rest of the day or are confident that you will remember to do them.

6. Finishing Touches: 5 minutes - End the day with a hot compress to heal any wear and tear and restore your penis to its previous, healthy state. This is, once again, an absolute must.
These six steps, when combined, form a healthy program that will not only help you address penis enhancement in any way you desire, but will also ensure that you do so in a healthy manner. The key is repetition: you will begin to see results fairly quickly, but serious results should be expected within a few months. You should aim to complete your full program at least five times per week, with the low impact speed workout only being used when absolutely necessary.
When your program is completed, you will have a longer and thicker penis, increased stamina to use it, and a much firmer erection. What more could you and your lover ask for?

Monitoring Your Progress

After all of this effort, you'll obviously want to keep a close eye on the length and girth of your penis to see how much you've already grown. We wouldn't blame you if you did this almost daily, but just as dieters are advised to avoid the scales outside of their weekly check-in, it's best to do a check no more than once a week. As a result, you will notice larger changes during each measure and will have a better understanding of how effective your work has been.

You should also always measure your penis in its fully erect position because, after all, that's what you're really interested in. According to research, there is no correlation between the size of your soft penis and its size while erect. Because there is such a distinction between a "grower" and a "shower," and the amount your penis grows when it becomes erect can range from almost nothing to four full inches, it's entirely possible that you won't notice the same difference in both states - so focus on the one that really matters.

The changes you want to see should be visible and tangible while your penis is in the state you'll be using it, so do your measuring then.

A Final Thought on Safety

We've mentioned it several times throughout the book, but it's so crucial to your overall well-being - both sexually and otherwise - that it bears repeating before we leave you to your exercises.

Before you begin any exercise, make certain that you have thoroughly read the instructions. Performing an exercise that requires lubricant without any or one that requires a flaccid penis with an erect one will, at the very least, prevent you from making the desired enhancement gains and, at worst, may result in long-term damage.
Don't go overboard, either. Growing your penis is not a one-day dream; it will require you to be patient and determined in your efforts over many weeks and months. It will be worthwhile in the end, so resist the urge to cram a year's worth of exercise into a single day if you still want to walk in the morning.

If you're frustrated by the slow results of these exercises, avoid risky alternatives. If you know ahead of time that you won't be measuring extra inches by the end of a week, you'll have a better chance of resisting the more sinister penis enhancement offers. Clamping yourself with metal, undergoing surgery, or using a machine to suck on your penis will not produce better results than your exercise regimen and may result in irreversible damage.

Finally, keep an eye out for any discomfort or pain during your sessions.
These don't always mean you should stop, and the instructions will tell you if they're normal to feel, but they can be a warning sign. If you are in pain, it is possible that you are performing the exercise incorrectly or that you have performed too many repetitions for your current comfort levels. You'll get far better results if you listen to your body.

Conclusion

We're thrilled to have brought you the real secrets of penis enhancement - reading the witchcraft and mad scientist options that are so readily available in the depths of the internet was starting to irritate us. We know from experience that these techniques will produce far better and healthier results than a pump or a shady pill bottle.

With these secrets in hand, we hope you'll embark on a journey to sexual fulfillment that will satisfy both you and your lovers. Your penis will not only be the length you've always desired, but it will also have the girth that so many women claim is important to their pleasure. Your penis will be loud and proud, with erections that are firm, strong, and long-lasting. As you establish and increase control over your penis, you will be able to control the pace and last as long as you want in the bedroom.

You'll be stronger, more confident, and more than a little eager to get out there and test the results by the time you see extra inches on the tape measure.
You'll know you have everything you need to become a bedroom legend, and you'll never again avoid talking to the man or woman of your dreams for fear of being disappointed by the size of your package or what you can do with it.

People always say that size isn't everything, and we partially agree.
The truth is that size is only one component of the overall picture, and it is useless without strength, stamina, and confidence. To be the full package, you must have the full package, which you can now have thanks to this program.

www.ingramcontent.com/pod-product-compliance
Ingram Content Group UK Ltd.
Pitfield, Milton Keynes, MK11 3LW, UK
UKHW061706190726
13853UKWH00008B/2422

9 798393 087937